Keto Air Fryer Meat Recipes

Stay Healthy and Fit with These Tasty Recipes

Lydia Gorman

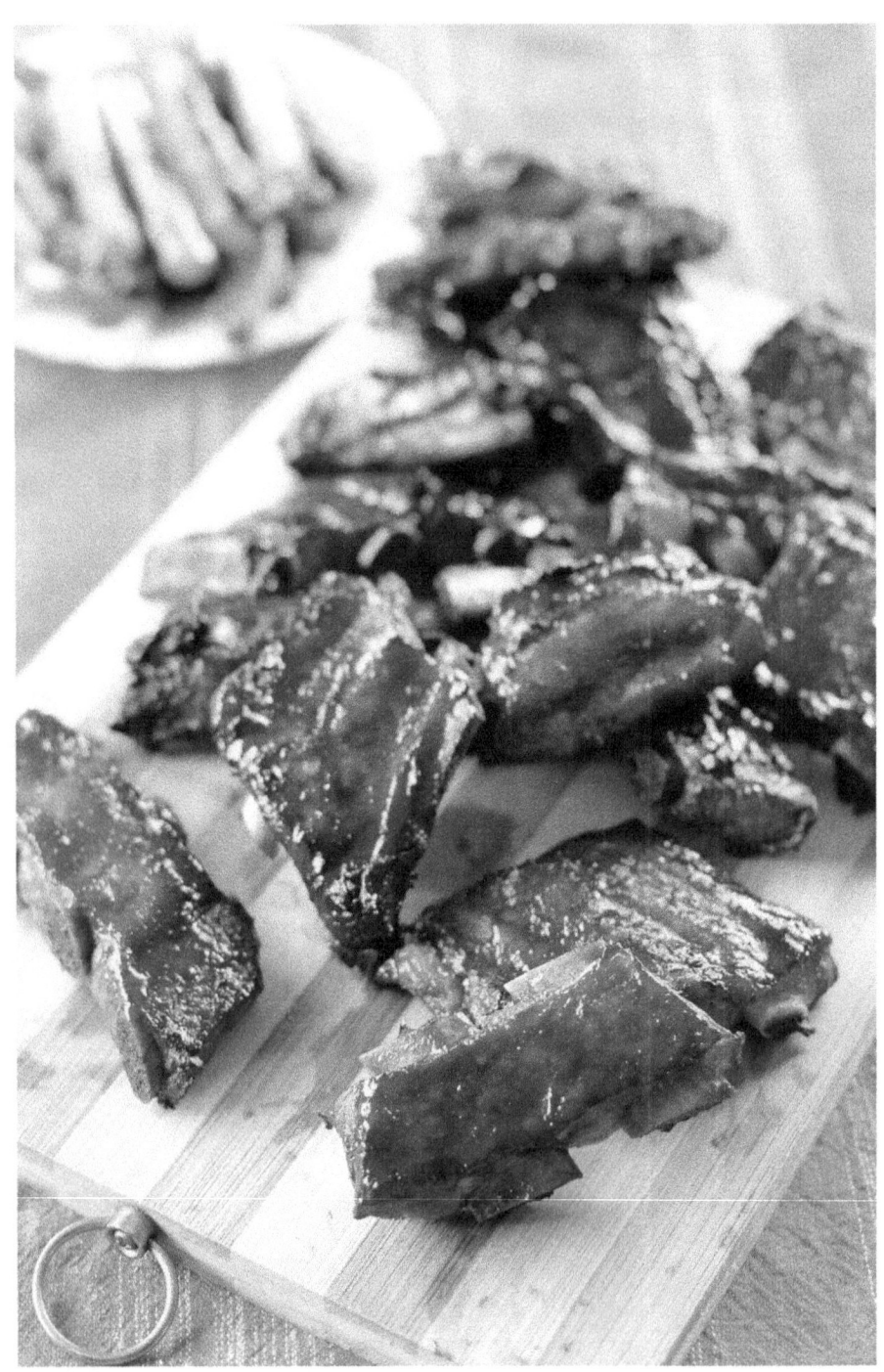

© Copyright 2020 All rights reserved.

The following Book is reproduced below with the goal of providing information that is as accurate and reliable as possible. Regardless, purchasing this Book can be seen as consent to the fact that both the publisher and the author of this book are in no way experts on the topics discussed within and that any recommendations or suggestions that are made herein are for entertainment purposes only. Professionals should be consulted as needed prior to undertaking any of the action endorsed herein.

This declaration is deemed fair and valid by both the American Bar Association and the Committee of Publishers Association and is legally binding throughout the United States.

Furthermore, the transmission, duplication, or reproduction of any of the following work including specific information will be considered an illegal act irrespective of

if it is done electronically or in print. This extends to creating a secondary or tertiary copy of the work or a recorded copy and is only allowed with the express written consent from the Publisher. All additional right reserved.

The information in the following pages is broadly considered a truthful and accurate account of facts and as such, any inattention, use, or misuse of the information in question by the reader will render any resulting actions solely under their purview. There are no scenarios in which the publisher or the original author of this work can be in any fashion deemed liable for any hardship or damages that may befall them after undertaking information described herein.

Additionally, the information in the following pages is intended only for informational purposes and should thus be thought of as universal. As befitting its nature, it is presented without assurance regarding its prolonged validity or interim quality. Trademarks that are mentioned are done without written consent and can in no way be considered an endorsement from the trademark holder.

Table of Contents

SIMPLE & JUICY STEAK 9
PORK CHOP FRIES 11
SPICY PORK PATTIES 14
SPICY PARMESAN PORK CHOPS 16
AIR FRIED PORK BITES 18
STEAK TIPS 20
RANCH PATTIES 22
EASY BEEF KEBABS 24
AIR FRYER BEEF FAJITAS 26
JUICY PORK TENDERLOIN 29
LEMON PEPPER PORK 31
STUFFED PORK CHOPS 32
AIR FRYER LAMB CHOPS 34
BREADED PORK CHOPS 36
CREOLE SEASONED PORK CHOPS 38
COCONUT PORK CHOPS 40
JERK PORK CUBES 42
SMOKEY STEAKS 44
SIMPLE BEEF KABAB 46
SPICY PORK TENDERLOIN 48
GARLIC THYME LAMB CHOPS 50
DELICIOUS HERB BEEF PATTIES 52
ROASTED SIRLOIN STEAK 54
BASIL CHEESE LAMB PATTIES 56

AIR FRYER STEW MEAT	58
RANCH PORK CHOPS	60
TACO STUFFED PEPPERS	61
GARLICKY PORK CHOPS	63
DIJON PORK CHOPS	65
PECAN DIJON PORK CHOPS	67
MARINATED RIBEYE STEAKS	69
PORK KEBABS	71
HERB PORK CHOPS	73
PORK CHOPS	75
BEEF KEBABS	77
ROSEMARY BEEF TIPS	79
SIRLOIN STEAK	81
STEAK & MUSHROOMS	83
FLAVORFUL BURGER PATTIES	85
BAKED BEEF & BROCCOLI	87
SPICED PORK TENDERLOIN	89
SPICY PORK CHOPS	91
LEMON HERB LAMB CHOPS	93
CAJUN HERB PORK CHOPS	95
THAI PORK CHOPS	97
SAVORY DASH SEASONED PORK CHOPS	99
SPICY ASIAN LAMB	100
CHIPOTLE STEAK	102
BAKED LAMB CHOPS	104
LEMON GARLIC SIRLOIN STEAK	106

Introduction

What's the difference between an air fryer and deep fryer? Air fryers bake food at a high temperature with a high-powered fan, while deep fryers cook food in a vat of oil that has been heated up to a specific temperature. Both cook food quickly, but an air fryer requires practically zero preheat time while a deep fryer can take upwards of 10 minutes. Air fryers also require little to no oil and deep fryers require a lot that absorb into the food. Food comes out crispy and juicy in both appliances, but don't taste the same, usually because deep fried foods are coated in batter that cook differently in an air fryer vs a deep fryer. Battered foods needs to be sprayed with oil before cooking in an air fryer to help them color and get crispy, while the hot oil soaks into the batter in a deep fryer. Flour-based batters and wet batters don't cook well in an air fryer, but they come out very well in a deep fryer.

The ketogenic diet is one such example. The diet calls for a very small number of carbs to be eaten. This means food such as rice, pasta, and other starchy vegetables like potatoes are off the menu. Even relaxed versions of the keto diet minimize carbs to a large extent and this compromises the goals of many dieters. They end up having to exert large amounts of willpower to follow the diet. This doesn't do them any favors since willpower is like a muscle. At some point, it tires and this is when the dieter goes right back to their old pattern of eating. I have personal experience with this. In terms of health benefits, the keto diet offers the most. The reduction of carbs forces your body to mobilize fat and this results in automatic fat loss and better health.

Feel free to mix and match the recipes you see in here and play around with them. Eating is supposed to be fun! Unfortunately, we've associated fun eating with unhealthy food. This doesn't have to be the case. The air fryer, combined with the Mediterranean diet, will make your mealtimes fun-filled again and full of taste. There's no grease and messy cleanups to deal with anymore. Are you excited yet?

You should be! You're about to embark on a journey full of air fried goodness!

Simple & Juicy Steak

Preparation Time: 10 minutes

Cooking Time: 13 minutes

Serve: 2

Ingredients:

12 oz ribeye steak

1 tsp steak seasoning

1 tbsp olive oil

Pepper

Salt

Directions:

Coat steak with oil and season with steak seasoning, pepper, and salt.

Place the cooking tray in the air fryer basket.

Select Air Fry mode.

Set time to 13 minutes and temperature 400 F then press START.

The air fryer display will prompt you to ADD FOOD once the temperature is reached then place steak in the air fryer basket.

Serve and enjoy.

Pork Chop Fries

Preparation Time: 10 minutes

Cooking Time: 15 minutes

Serve: 4

Ingredients:

1lb pork chops, cut into fries

1/2 cup parmesan cheese, grated

3.5 oz pork rinds, crushed

1/2 cup ranch dressing

Pepper

Salt

Directions:

In a shallow dish, mix together crushed pork rinds, parmesan cheese, pepper, and salt.

Add pork chop pieces and ranch dressing into the zip-lock bag, seal bag, and shake well.

Remove pork chop pieces from zip-lock bag and coat with crushed pork rind mixture.

Place the cooking tray in the air fryer basket.

Line air fryer basket with parchment paper.

Select Bake mode.

Set time to 15 minutes and temperature 400 F then press START.

The air fryer display will prompt you to ADD FOOD once the temperature is reached then place breaded pork chop fries in the air fryer basket.

Serve and enjoy.

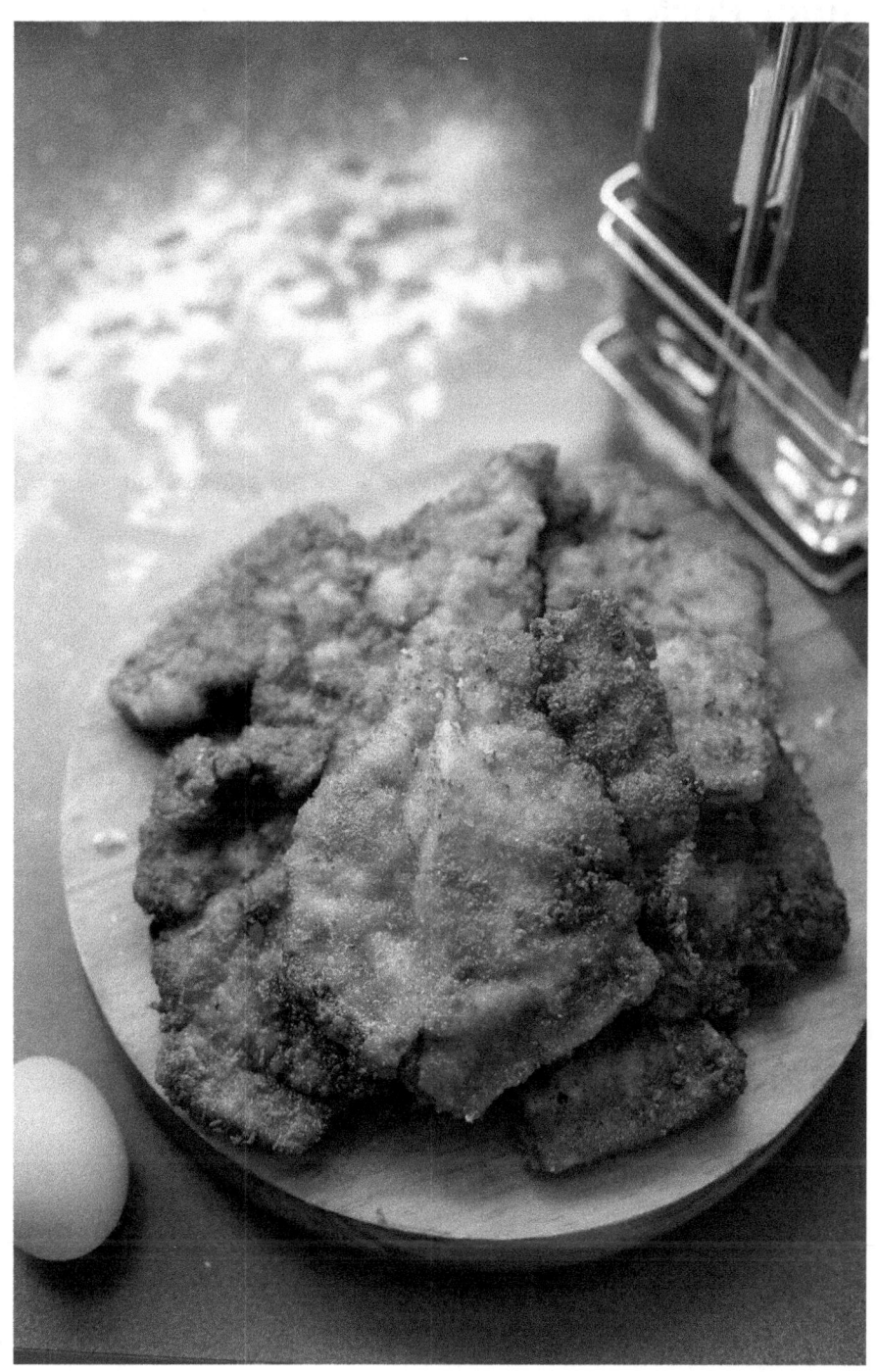

Spicy Pork Patties

Preparation Time: 10 minutes

Cooking Time: 10 minutes

Serve: 2

Ingredients:

1/2 lb ground pork

1 tbsp Cajun seasoning

1 egg, lightly beaten

1/2 cup almond flour

Pepper

Salt

Directions:

Add all ingredients into the large bowl and mix until well combined.

Make two equal shapes of patties from the meat mixture.

Select Air Fry mode.

Set time to 10 minutes and temperature 360 F then press START.

The air fryer display will prompt you to ADD FOOD once the temperature is reached then place patties in the air fryer basket.

Serve and enjoy.

Spicy Parmesan Pork Chops

Preparation Time: 10 minutes

Cooking Time: 9 minutes

Serve: 2

Ingredients:

2 pork chops, boneless

1 tsp paprika

3 tbsp parmesan cheese, grated

1/3 cup almond flour

1 tsp Cajun seasoning

1 tsp dried mixed herbs

Directions:

In a shallow bowl, mix together parmesan cheese, almond flour, paprika, mixed herbs, and Cajun seasoning.

Spray pork chops with cooking spray and coat with parmesan cheese.

Select Air Fry mode.

Set time to 9 minutes and temperature 350 F then press START.

The air fryer display will prompt you to ADD FOOD once the temperature is reached then place breaded pork chops in the air fryer basket.

Turn pork chops halfway through. Serve and enjoy.

Air Fried Pork Bites

Preparation Time: 10 minutes

Cooking Time: 15 minutes

Serve: 4

Ingredients:

1 lb pork belly, cut into 1-inch cubes

1 tsp soy sauce

Pepper

Salt

Directions:

In a bowl, toss pork cubes with soy sauce, pepper, and salt.

Select Air Fry mode.

Set time to 15 minutes and temperature 400 F then press START.

The air fryer display will prompt you to ADD FOOD once the temperature is reached then place pork cubes in the air fryer basket.

Serve and enjoy.

Steak Tips

Preparation Time: 10 minutes

Cooking Time: 5 minutes

Serve: 3

Ingredients:

1 lb steak, cut into cubes

1 tsp olive oil

1 tsp Montreal steak seasoning

Pepper

Salt

Directions:

In a bowl, add steak cubes and remaining ingredients and toss well.

Select Air Fry mode.

Set time to 5 minutes and temperature 400 F then press START.

The air fryer display will prompt you to ADD FOOD once the temperature is reached then place steak cubes in the air fryer basket.

Serve and enjoy.

Ranch Patties

Preparation Time: 10 minutes

Cooking Time: 12 minutes

Serve: 4

Ingredients:

1 lb ground beef

1/2 tsp dried dill

1/2 tsp onion powder

1/2 tsp garlic powder

2 tsp dried parsley

1/8 tsp dried dill

1/2 tsp paprika

Pepper

Salt

Directions:

Add all ingredients into the large bowl and mix until well combined.

Make 4 even shape patties from meat mixture.

Select Air Fry mode.

Set time to 12 minutes and temperature 350 F then press START.

The air fryer display will prompt you to ADD FOOD once the temperature is reached then place patties in the air fryer basket.

Serve and enjoy.

Easy Beef Kebabs

Preparation Time: 10 minutes

Cooking Time: 10 minutes

Serve: 4

Ingredients:

1 lb beef chuck ribs, cut into 1-inch pieces

1/2 onion, cut into 1-inch pieces

2 tbsp soy sauce

1/3 cup sour cream

1 bell pepper, cut into 1-inch pieces

Directions:

Add meat pieces, soy sauce, and sour cream into the mixing bowl and mix well.

Cover bowl and place in the refrigerator overnight.

Thread marinated meat, onion, and bell peppers pieces onto the soaked wooden skewers.

Select Air Fry mode. Set time to 10 minutes and temperature 400 F then press START.

The air fryer display will prompt you to ADD FOOD once the temperature is reached then place skewers in the air fryer basket.

Turn halfway through.

Serve and enjoy.

Air Fryer Beef Fajitas

Preparation Time: 10 minutes

Cooking Time: 8 minutes

Serve: 4

Ingredients:

1 lb steak, sliced

1/2 tbsp chili powder

3 tbsp olive oil

2 bell peppers, sliced

1 tsp garlic powder

1 tsp paprika

1 tsp cumin

Pepper

Salt

Directions:

In a mixing bowl, toss sliced steak with remaining ingredients.

Select Air Fry mode.

Set time to 8 minutes and temperature 390 F then press START.

The air fryer display will prompt you to ADD FOOD once the temperature is reached then place fajitas in the air fryer basket.

Serve and enjoy.

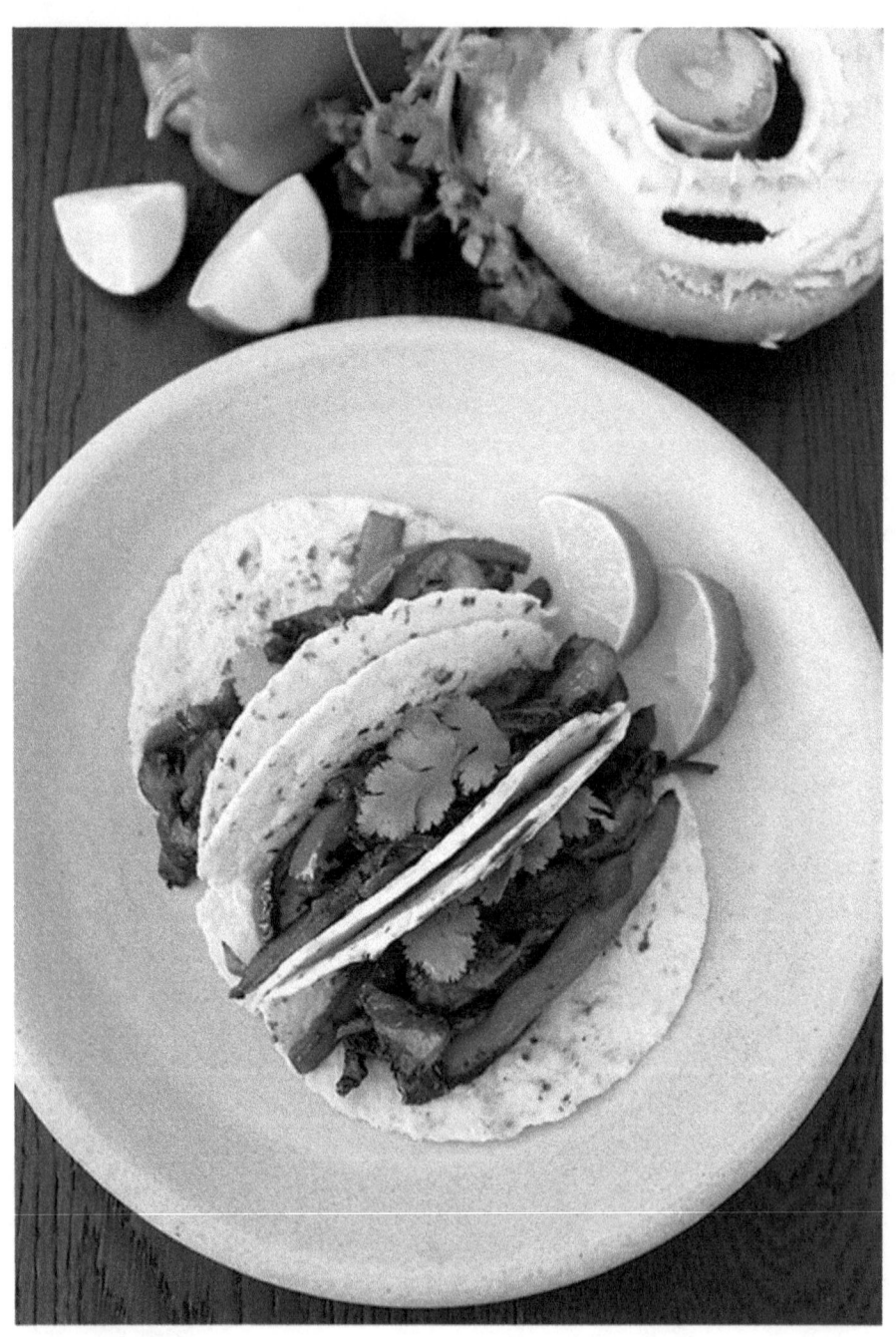

Juicy Pork Tenderloin

Preparation Time: 10 minutes

Cooking Time: 20 minutes

Serve: 4

Ingredients:

1 1/2 lbs pork tenderloin

2 tbsp olive oil

1 tsp garlic powder

1 tsp Italian seasoning

1/4 tsp pepper

1 tsp sea salt

Directions:

Rub pork tenderloin with 1 tablespoon of olive oil.

Mix together garlic powder, Italian seasoning, pepper, and salt and rub over pork tenderloin.

Heat remaining oil in a pan over medium-high heat.

Add pork tenderloin in hot oil and cook until brown Select Bake mode.

Set time to 15 minutes and temperature 400 F then press START.

The air fryer display will prompt you to ADD FOOD once the temperature is reached then place pork tenderloin in the air fryer basket.

Serve and enjoy.

Lemon Pepper Pork

Preparation Time: 10 minutes

Cooking Time: 15 minutes

Serve: 4

Ingredients:

4 pork chops, boneless

1 tsp lemon pepper seasoning

Salt

Directions:

Season pork chops with lemon pepper seasoning, and salt.

Select Air Fry mode.

Set time to 15 minutes and temperature 400 F then press START.

The air fryer display will prompt you to ADD FOOD once the temperature is reached then place pork chops in the air fryer basket.

Serve and enjoy.

Stuffed Pork Chops

Preparation Time: 10 minutes

Cooking Time: 35 minutes

Serve: 4

Ingredients:

4 pork chops, boneless and thick-cut

2 tbsp olives, chopped

2 tbsp sun-dried tomatoes, chopped

1/2 cup feta cheese, crumbled

2 garlic cloves, minced

2 tbsp fresh parsley, chopped

Directions:

In a bowl, combine together feta cheese, garlic, parsley, olives, and sun-dried tomatoes.

Stuff cheese mixture all the pork chops.

Season pork chops with pepper and salt.

Select Bake mode.

Set time to 35 minutes and temperature 375 F then press START.

The air fryer display will prompt you to ADD FOOD once the temperature is reached then place stuffed pork chops in the air fryer basket.

Serve and enjoy

Air Fryer Lamb Chops

Preparation Time: 10 minutes

Cooking Time: 12 minutes

Serve: 4

Ingredients:

4 lamb chops

2 garlic clove, minced

3 tbsp olive oil

Pepper

Salt

Directions:

In a small bowl, mix together thyme and oil.

Season lamb chops with pepper and salt and rubs with thyme mixture.

Select Air Fry mode.

Set time to 12 minutes and temperature 400 F then press START.

The air fryer display will prompt you to ADD FOOD once the temperature is reached then place lamb chops in the air fryer basket.

Turn halfway through.

Serve and enjoy.

Breaded Pork Chops

Preparation Time: 10 minutes

Cooking Time: 20 minutes

Serve: 4

Ingredients:

4 pork chops, boneless

1/4 cup parmesan cheese, grated

1 cup almond meal

1/2 tbsp black pepper

1 tbsp onion powder

1 tbsp garlic powder

2 eggs, lightly beaten

1/2 tsp sea salt

Directions:

In a bowl, mix together almond meal, parmesan cheese, onion powder, garlic powder, pepper, and salt.

Whisk eggs in a shallow dish.

Dip pork chops into the egg then coat with almond meal mixture.

Select Air Fry mode.

Set time to 20 minutes and temperature 350 F then press START.

The air fryer display will prompt you to ADD FOOD once the temperature is reached then place breaded pork chops in the air fryer basket.

Turn pork chops halfway through.

Serve and enjoy.

Creole Seasoned Pork Chops

Preparation Time: 10 minutes

Cooking Time: 12 minutes

Serve: 6

Ingredients:

1 1/2 lbs pork chops, boneless

1/4 cup parmesan cheese, grated

1/3 cup almond flour

1 tsp paprika

1 tsp Creole seasoning

1 tsp garlic powder

Directions:

Add all ingredients except pork chops into the zip-lock bag.

Add pork chops into the bag. Seal bag and shake well.

Remove pork chops from the zip-lock bag.

Select Air Fry mode.

Set time to 12 minutes and temperature 360 F then press START.

The air fryer display will prompt you to ADD FOOD once the temperature is reached then place pork chops in the air fryer basket.

Serve and enjoy.

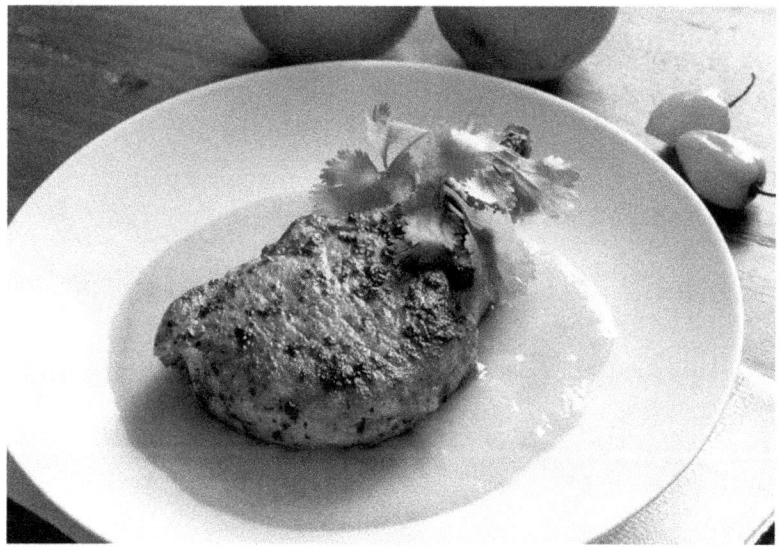

Coconut Pork Chops

Preparation Time: 10 minutes

Cooking Time: 14 minutes

Serve: 4

Ingredients:

4 pork chops

1 tbsp coconut oil

1 tbsp coconut butter

2 tsp parsley

2 tsp garlic, grated

Pepper

Salt

Directions:

In a large bowl, mix together with seasonings, garlic, butter, and coconut oil.

Add pork chops to the bowl and mix well.

Place in refrigerator overnight.

Select Air Fry mode.

Set time to 14 minutes and temperature 350 F then press START.

The air fryer display will prompt you to ADD FOOD once the temperature is reached then place marinated pork chops in the air fryer basket.

Turn pork chops halfway through. Serve and enjoy.

Jerk Pork Cubes

Preparation Time: 10 minutes

Cooking Time: 20 minutes

Serve: 4

Ingredients:

1 1/2 lbs pork butt, cut into pieces

1/4 cup jerk paste

Pepper

Salt

Directions:

Add meat and jerk paste into the bowl and mix well and place in refrigerator overnight.

Select Air Fry mode.

Set time to 20 minutes and temperature 390 F then press START.

The air fryer display will prompt you to ADD FOOD once the temperature is reached then place marinated pork pieces in the air fryer basket.

Stir halfway through.

Serve and enjoy.

Smokey Steaks

Preparation Time: 10 minutes

Cooking Time: 7 minutes

Serve: 2

Ingredients:

12 oz steaks

1 tbsp Montreal steak seasoning

1 tsp liquid smoke

1 tbsp soy sauce

1/2 tbsp cocoa powder

Pepper

Salt

Directions:

Add steak, liquid smoke, soy sauce, and steak seasonings into the large zip-lock bag.

Shake well and place it in the refrigerator overnight.

Select Air Fry mode.

Set time to 7 minutes and temperature 375 F then press START.

The air fryer display will prompt you to ADD FOOD once the temperature is reached then place steaks in the air fryer basket.

Turn steaks after 5 minutes.

Serve and enjoy.

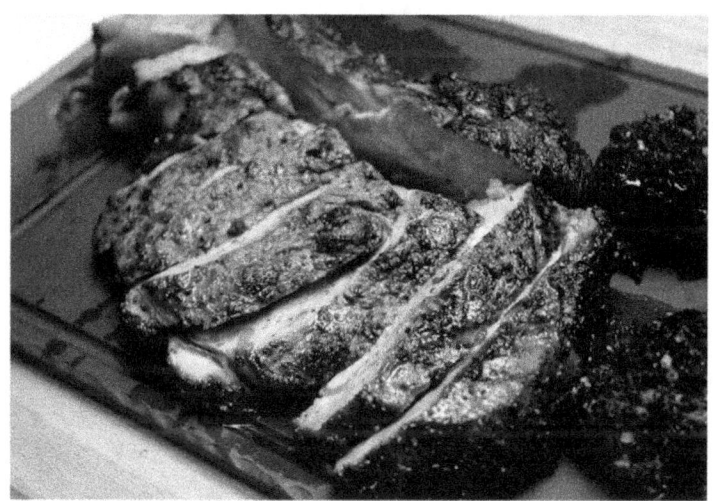

Simple Beef Kabab

Preparation Time: 10 minutes

Cooking Time: 10 minutes

Serve: 4

Ingredients:

1lb ground beef

2 tbsp kabab spice mix

1 tbsp garlic, minced

1 tbsp olive oil

1 tsp salt

Directions:

Add all ingredients into the mixing bowl and mix until well combined.

Place in refrigerator for 30 minutes.

Divide mixture into the 4 equal portions and make sausage shape kabab.

Select Air Fry mode.

Set time to 10 minutes and temperature 370 F then press START.

The air fryer display will prompt you to ADD FOOD once the temperature is reached then place kabab in the air fryer basket.

Serve and enjoy.

Spicy Pork Tenderloin

Preparation Time: 10 minutes

Cooking Time: 35 minutes

Serve: 6

Ingredients:

2 pork tenderloin

For rub:

1 tbsp smoked paprika

1 tbsp garlic powder

1 tbsp onion powder

1/2 tbsp salt

Directions:

In a small bowl, combine together all rub ingredients.

Coat pork tenderloin with the rub.

Heat ovenproof pan over medium-high heat.

Spray pan with cooking spray.

Sear pork on all sides until lightly golden brown.

Select Bake mode.

Set time to 30 minutes and temperature 400 F then press START.

The air fryer display will prompt you to ADD FOOD once the temperature is reached then place pork tenderloin in the air fryer basket.

Serve and enjoy.

Garlic Thyme Lamb Chops

Preparation Time: 5 minutes

Cooking Time: 12 minutes

Serve: 4

Ingredients:

4 lamb chops

4 garlic clove, minced

3 tbsp olive oil

Pepper

Salt

Directions:

In a small bowl, mix together oil and garlic.

Season lamb chops with pepper and salt and rubs with oil and garlic mixture.

Select Bake mode.

Set time to 12 minutes and temperature 400 F then press START.

The air fryer display will prompt you to ADD FOOD once the temperature is reached then place lamb chops in the air fryer basket.

Turn lamb chops halfway through.

Serve and enjoy.

Delicious Herb Beef Patties

Preparation Time: 10 minutes

Cooking Time: 45 minutes

Serve: 4

Ingredients:

10 oz beef minced

1/4 tsp ginger paste

1 1/2 tsp mixed herbs

1 tsp basil

1 tsp tomato puree

1 tsp garlic puree

1/2 tsp mustard

Pepper

Salt

Directions:

Add all ingredients into the large bowl and mix until well combined.

Make patties from meat mixture.

Select Air Fry mode.

Set time to 45 minutes and temperature 375 F then press START.

The air fryer display will prompt you to ADD FOOD once the temperature is reached then place patties in the air fryer basket.

Serve and enjoy.

Roasted Sirloin Steak

Preparation Time: 10 minutes

Cooking Time: 30 minutes

Serve: 6

Ingredients:

2 lbs sirloin steak, cut into 1-inch cubes

2 garlic cloves, minced

3 tbsp fresh lemon juice

1 tsp dried oregano

1/4 tsp thyme

1/4 cup water

1/4 cup olive oil

2 cups fresh parsley, chopped

1/2 tsp pepper

1 tsp salt

Directions:

Add all ingredients except beef into the large bowl and mix well.

Pour bowl mixture into the large zip-lock bag.

Add steak cubes into the bag and seal bag and place in refrigerator for 1 hour.

Place marinated beef on a baking dish and cover dish with foil.

Select Bake mode.

Set time to 30 minutes and temperature 400 F then press START.

The air fryer display will prompt you to ADD FOOD once the temperature is reached then place the baking dish in the air fryer basket.

Serve and enjoy.

Basil Cheese Lamb Patties

Preparation Time: 10 minutes

Cooking Time: 8 minutes

Serve: 4

Ingredients:

1 lb ground lamb

1 cup goat cheese, crumbled

1 tbsp garlic, minced

6 basil leaves, minced

1 tsp chili powder

1/4 cup mint leaves, minced

1/4 cup fresh parsley, chopped

1 tsp dried oregano

1/4 tsp pepper

1/2 tsp kosher salt

Directions:

Add all ingredients into the mixing bowl and mix until well combined.

Make four equal shape patties from the meat mixture.

Select Bake mode.

Set time to 8 minutes and temperature 400 F then press START.

The air fryer display will prompt you to ADD FOOD once the temperature is reached then place patties in the air fryer basket.

Turn patties halfway through.

Serve and enjoy.

Air Fryer Stew Meat

Preparation Time: 10 minutes

Cooking Time: 25 minutes

Serve: 4

Ingredients:

1 lb beef stew meat, cut into strips

1/2 lime juice

1 tbsp olive oil

1/2 tbsp ground cumin

1 tbsp garlic powder

1/2 tsp onion powder

Pepper

Salt

Directions:

Add meat and remaining ingredients into the mixing bowl and mix well.

Select Air Fry mode.

Set time to 25 minutes and temperature 380 F then press START.

The air fryer display will prompt you to ADD FOOD once the temperature is reached then place stew meat in the air fryer basket.

Stir halfway through Serve and enjoy.

Ranch Pork Chops

Preparation Time: 10 minutes

Cooking Time: 35 minutes

Serve: 4

Ingredients:

4 pork chops, boneless

1 oz ranch seasoning

1 1/2 tbsp olive oil

Directions:

Brush pork chops with oil and rub with ranch seasoning.

Select Air Fry mode.

Set time to 35 minutes and temperature 400 F then press START.

The air fryer display will prompt you to ADD FOOD once the temperature is reached then place pork chops in the air fryer basket.

Serve and enjoy.

Taco Stuffed Peppers

Preparation Time: 10 minutes

Cooking Time: 8 minutes

Serve: 12

Ingredients:

6 jalapeno peppers, cut in half & remove seeds

1 1/2 tbsp taco seasoning

1/2 lb ground beef

1/4 cup goat cheese, crumbled

Directions:

Browned the meat in a large pan.

Remove pan from heat.

Add taco seasoning to the ground meat and mix well.

Stuff meat into each jalapeno half.

Select Air Fry mode.

Set time to 6 minutes and temperature 320 F then press START.

The air fryer display will prompt you to ADD FOOD once the temperature is reached then place jalapeno halves in the air fryer basket.

Sprinkle cheese on top of peppers and cook for 2 minutes more. Serve and enjoy.

Garlicky Pork Chops

Preparation Time: 10 minutes

Cooking Time: 20 minutes

Serve: 8

Ingredients:

8 pork chops, boneless

6 garlic cloves, minced

1/4 tsp pepper

3/4 cup parmesan cheese

2 tbsp butter, melted

2 tbsp coconut oil

1 tsp thyme

1 tbsp parsley

1/2 tsp sea salt

Directions:

In a small bowl, mix together butter, garlic, pepper, thyme, parsley, parmesan cheese, coconut oil, and salt.

Brush butter mixture on top of pork chops.

Select Air Fry mode.

Set time to 20 minutes and temperature 400 F then press START.

The air fryer display will prompt you to ADD FOOD once the temperature is reached then place pork chops in the air fryer basket.

Turn pork chops halfway through.

Serve and enjoy.

Dijon Pork Chops

Preparation Time: 10 minutes

Cooking Time: 12 minutes

Serve: 4

Ingredients:

4 pork chops

1 tbsp garlic, minced

4 tbsp Dijon mustard

Pepper

Salt

Directions:

In a small bowl, mix together mustard, garlic, pepper, and salt Brush pork chops with mustard mixture.

Select Air Fry mode.

Set time to 12 minutes and temperature 350 F then press START.

The air fryer display will prompt you to ADD FOOD once the temperature is reached then place pork chops in the air fryer basket.

Turn pork chops halfway through.

Serve and enjoy.

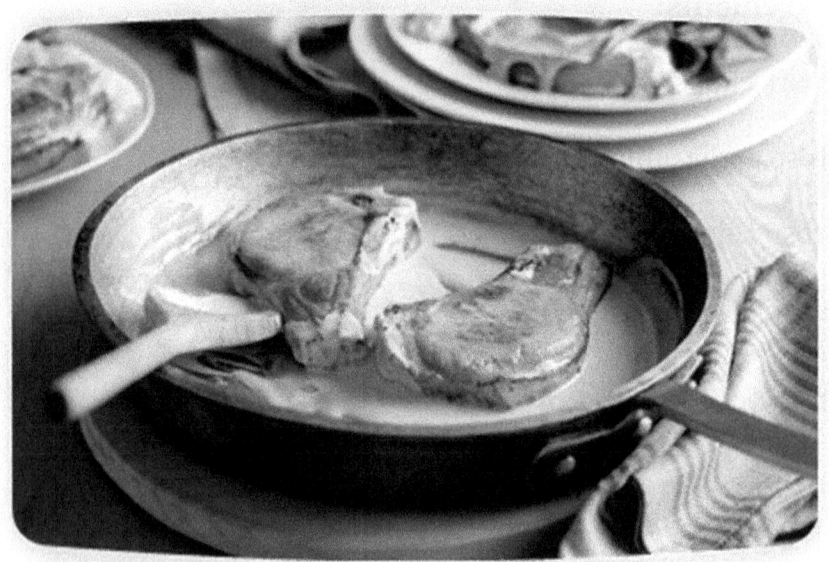

Pecan Dijon Pork Chops

Preparation Time: 10 minutes

Cooking Time: 12 minutes

Serve: 6

Ingredients:

1 egg

6 pork chops, boneless

2 garlic cloves, minced

1 tbsp water

1 tsp Dijon mustard

1 tsp garlic powder

1 tsp onion powder

2 tsp Italian seasoning

1/3 cup arrowroot

1 cup pecans, finely chopped

1/4 tsp salt

Directions:

In a shallow bowl, whisk the egg with garlic, water, and Dijon mustard.

In a separate shallow bowl, mix together arrowroot, pecans, Italian seasoning, onion powder, garlic powder, and salt.

Dip pork chop in the egg mixture and coat with arrowroot mixture.

Place the cooking tray in the air fryer basket.

Select Air Fry mode.

Set time to 12 minutes and temperature 400 F then press START.

The air fryer display will prompt you to ADD FOOD once the temperature is reached then place coated pork chops in the air fryer basket.

Turn pork chops halfway through.

Serve and enjoy.

Marinated Ribeye Steaks

Preparation Time: 10 minutes

Cooking Time: 12 minutes

Serve: 4

Ingredients:

2 large ribeye steaks,

1 1/2-inch thick

1 1/2 tbsp Montreal steak seasoning

1/2 cup low-sodium soy sauce

1/4 cup olive oil

Directions:

Add soy sauce, oil, and Montreal steak seasoning in a large zip-lock bag.

Add steaks in a zip-lock bag.

Seal bag shakes well and places in the refrigerator for 2 hours.

Place the cooking tray in the air fryer basket.

Select Air Fry mode.

Set time to 12 minutes and temperature 400 F then press START.

The air fryer display will prompt you to ADD FOOD once the temperature is reached then remove steaks from marinade and place in the air fryer basket.

Turn steaks halfway through. Serve and enjoy.

Pork Kebabs

Preparation Time: 10 minutes

Cooking Time: 15 minutes

Serve: 6

Ingredients:

2 lbs country-style pork ribs, cut into cubes

1/4 cup soy sauce

1/2 cup olive oil

1 tbsp Italian seasoning

Directions:

Add soy sauce, oil, Italian seasoning, and pork cubes into the zip-lock bag, seal bag and place in the refrigerator for 4 hours.

Remove pork cubes from marinade and place the cubes on wooden skewers.

Place the cooking tray in the air fryer basket.

Line air fryer basket with parchment paper.

Select Bake mode.

Set time to 15 minutes and temperature 380 F then press START.

The air fryer display will prompt you to ADD FOOD once the temperature is reached then place pork skewers in the air fryer basket.

Serve and enjoy

Herb Pork Chops

Preparation Time: 10 minutes

Cooking Time: 15 minutes

Serve: 4

Ingredients:

4 pork chops

2 tsp oregano

2 tsp thyme

2 tsp sage

1 tsp garlic powder

1 tsp paprika

1 tsp rosemary

Pepper

Salt

Directions:

Spray pork chops with cooking spray.

Mix together garlic powder, paprika, rosemary, oregano, thyme, sage, pepper, and salt and rub over pork chops.

Select Air Fry mode.

Set time to 15 minutes and temperature 360 F then press START.

The air fryer display will prompt you to ADD FOOD once the temperature is reached then place pork chops in the air fryer basket.

Turn pork chops halfway through.

Serve and enjoy.

Pork Chops

Preparation Time: 10 minutes

Cooking Time: 14 minutes

Serve: 2

Ingredients:

2 pork chops

1 tsp paprika

1 tsp garlic powder

1 tsp olive oil

Pepper

Salt

Directions:

Brush pork chops with olive oil and season with garlic powder, paprika, pepper, and salt.

Select Air Fry mode.

Set time to 14 minutes and temperature 360 F then press START.

The air fryer display will prompt you to ADD FOOD once the temperature is reached then place pork chops in the air fryer basket.

Turn pork chops halfway through.

Beef Kebabs

Preparation Time: 10 minutes

Cooking Time: 15 minutes

Serve: 4

Ingredients:

1 lb ground beef

1/2 cup onion, minced

1/4 tsp ground cinnamon

1/4 tsp ground cardamom

1/2 tsp cayenne

1/2 tsp turmeric

1/2 tbsp ginger paste

1/2 tbsp garlic paste

1/4 cup cilantro, chopped

1 tsp salt

Directions:

Add meat and remaining ingredients into the large bowl and mix until well combined.

Make sausage shape kebabs.

Select Bake mode.

Set time to 15 minutes and temperature 350 F then press START.

The air fryer display will prompt you to ADD FOOD once the temperature is reached then place kebabs in the air fryer basket.

Serve and enjoy.

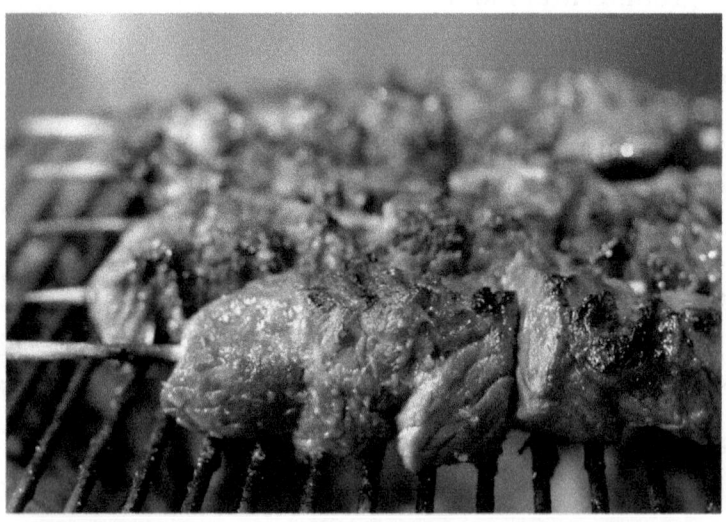

Rosemary Beef Tips

Preparation Time: 10 minutes

Cooking Time: 12 minutes

Serve: 4

Ingredients:

1 lb steak, cut into 1-inch cubes

1 tsp paprika

2 tsp onion powder

1 tsp garlic powder

2 tbsp coconut aminos

2 tsp rosemary, crushed

Pepper

Salt

Directions:

Add meat and remaining ingredients into the mixing bowl and mix well and let it sit for 5 minutes.

Select Air Fry mode.

Set time to 12 minutes and temperature 380 F then press START.

The air fryer display will prompt you to ADD FOOD once the temperature is reached then place steak cubes in the air fryer basket.

Stir halfway through.

Serve and enjoy.

Sirloin Steak

Preparation Time: 10 minutes

Cooking Time: 14 minutes

Serve: 2

Ingredients:

1 lb sirloin steaks

1/2 tsp garlic powder

1/4 tsp onion powder

1 tsp olive oil

Pepper

Salt

Directions:

Brush steak with olive oil and rub with garlic powder, onion powder, pepper, and salt.

Select Air Fry mode.

Set time to 14 minutes and temperature 400 F then press START.

The air fryer display will prompt you to ADD FOOD once the temperature is reached then place steaks in the air fryer basket.

Turn steak halfway through.

Serve and enjoy.

Steak & Mushrooms

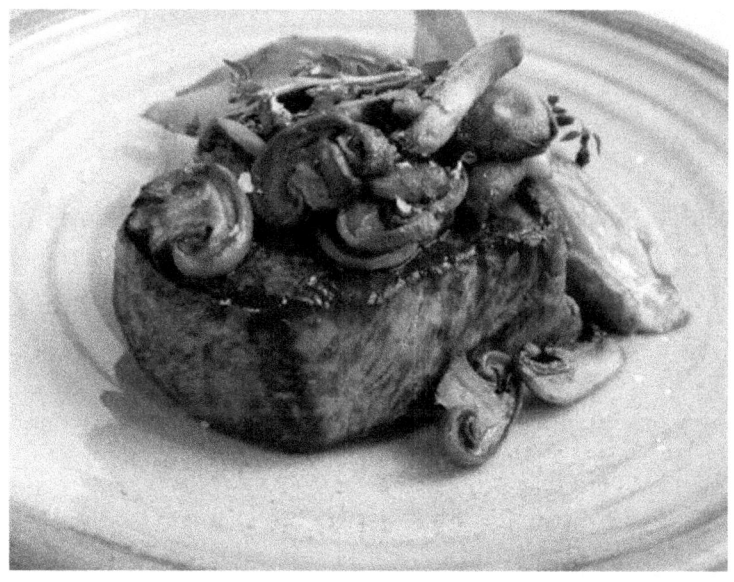

Preparation Time: 10 minutes

Cooking Time: 18 minutes

Serve: 4

Ingredients:

1 lb steaks, cut into 1-inch cubes

2 tbsp olive oil

8 oz mushrooms, halved

1/2 tsp garlic powder

1 tsp Worcestershire sauce

Pepper

Salt

Directions:

Add steak cubes and remaining ingredients into the mixing bowl and toss until well coated.

Select Air Fry mode.

Set time to 18 minutes and temperature 400 F then press START.

The air fryer display will prompt you to ADD FOOD once the temperature is reached then place steak and mushrooms in the air fryer basket.

Stir halfway through.

Serve and enjoy.

Flavorful Burger Patties

Preparation Time: 10 minutes

Cooking Time: 15 minutes

Serve: 4

Ingredients:

1 lb ground lamb

1/4 tsp cayenne pepper

1/4 cup fresh parsley, chopped

1/4 cup onion, minced

1 tbsp garlic, minced

1/2 tsp ground allspice

1 tsp ground cinnamon

1 tsp ground coriander

1 tsp ground cumin

1/4 tsp pepper

1 tsp kosher salt

Directions:

Add all ingredients into the large bowl and mix until well combined.

Make 4 patties from the meat mixture.

Select Bake mode.

Set time to 14 minutes and temperature 375 F then press START.

The air fryer display will prompt you to ADD FOOD once the temperature is reached then place patties in the air fryer basket.

Turn patties halfway through.

Serve and enjoy

Baked Beef & Broccoli

Preparation Time: 10 minutes

Cooking Time: 25 minutes

Serve: 2

Ingredients:

1/2 cup broccoli florets

1/2 lb beef stew meat, cut into pieces

1 onion, sliced

1 tbsp vinegar

1 tbsp olive oil

Pepper

Salt

Directions:

Add meat and remaining ingredients into the large bowl and toss well.

Select Bake mode.

Set time to 25 minutes and temperature 390 F then press START.

The air fryer display will prompt you to ADD FOOD once the temperature is reached then place beef and broccoli in the air fryer basket.

Serve and enjoy.

Spiced Pork Tenderloin

Preparation Time: 10 minutes

Cooking Time: 35 minutes

Serve: 6

Ingredients:

2 lbs pork tenderloin

For the spice mix:

1/2 tsp allspice

1 tsp cinnamon

1 tsp cumin

1 tsp coriander

1/4 tsp cayenne

1 tsp oregano

1/4 tsp cloves

Directions:

In a small bowl, mix together all spice ingredients and set aside.

Using a sharp knife make slits on pork tenderloin and insert chopped garlic into each slit.

Rub spice mixture over pork tenderloin.

Sprinkle with pepper and salt.

Select Bake mode.

Set time to 35 minutes and temperature 375 F then press START.

The air fryer display will prompt you to ADD FOOD once the temperature is reached then place pork tenderloin in the air fryer basket.

Serve and enjoy.

Spicy Pork Chops

Preparation Time: 10 minutes

Cooking Time: 10 minutes

Serve: 4

Ingredients:

4 pork chops

1/2 tsp black pepper

1/2 tsp ground cumin

1 1/2 tsp olive oil

1/2 tsp dried sage

1 tsp cayenne pepper

1 tsp paprika

1/2 tsp garlic salt

Directions:

In a small bowl, mix together paprika, garlic salt, sage, pepper, cayenne pepper, and cumin.

Rub pork chops with spice mixture.

Spray pork chops with cooking spray.

Select Bake mode.

Set time to 10 minutes and temperature 400 F then press START.

The air fryer display will prompt you to ADD FOOD once the temperature is reached then place pork chops in the air fryer basket.

Turn pork chops halfway through.

Serve and enjoy.

Lemon Herb Lamb Chops

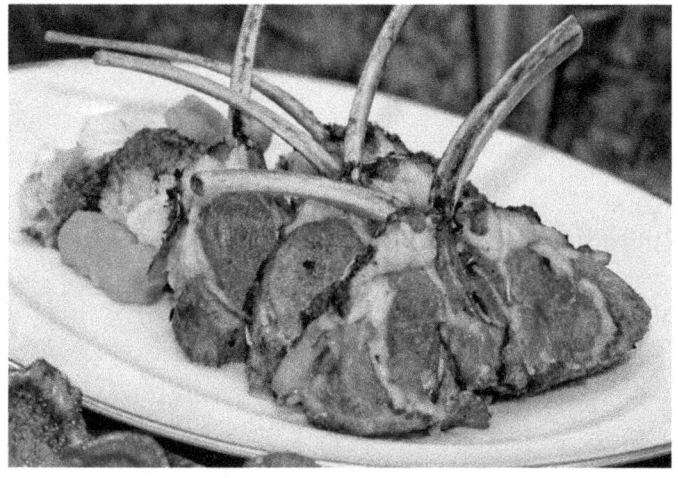

Preparation Time: 10 minutes

Cooking Time: 16 minutes

Serve: 4

Ingredients:

1lb lamb chops

1 tsp coriander

1 tsp oregano

1 tsp thyme

1 tsp rosemary

2 tbsp fresh lemon juice

2 tbsp olive oil

1 tsp salt

Directions:

Add all ingredients except lamb chops into the zip-lock bag.

Add lamb chops to the bag.

Seal bag and place in the refrigerator overnight.

Select Air Fry mode. Set time to 16 minutes and temperature 390 F then press START.

The air fryer display will prompt you to ADD FOOD once the temperature is reached then place lamb chops in the air fryer basket.

Turn lamb chops halfway through.

Serve and enjoy.

Cajun Herb Pork Chops

Preparation Time: 10 minutes

Cooking Time: 9 minutes

Serve: 2

Ingredients:

2 pork chops, boneless

1 tsp herb de Provence

1 tsp paprika

1/2 tsp Cajun seasoning

3 tbsp parmesan cheese, grated

1/3 cup almond flour

Directions:

Mix together almond flour, Cajun seasoning, herb de Provence, paprika, and parmesan cheese.

Spray both the pork chops with cooking spray.

Coat both the pork chops with almond flour mixture.

Select Bake mode.

Set time to 8 minutes and temperature 350 F then press START.

The air fryer display will prompt you to ADD FOOD once the temperature is reached then place pork chops in the air fryer basket.

Turn pork chops halfway through.

Serve and enjoy.

Thai Pork Chops

Preparation Time: 10 minutes

Cooking Time: 12 minutes

Serve: 2

Ingredients:

2 pork chops

1 tsp black pepper

3 tbsp lemongrass, chopped

1 tbsp shallot, chopped

1 tbsp garlic, chopped

1 tsp liquid stevia

1 tbsp sesame oil

1 tbsp fish sauce

1 tsp soy sauce

Directions:

Add pork chops in a mixing bowl.

Pour remaining ingredients over the pork chops and mix well.

Place in refrigerator for 2 hours.

Select Air Fry mode.

Set time to 12 minutes and temperature 400 F then press START.

The air fryer display will prompt you to ADD FOOD once the temperature is reached then place marinated pork chops in the air fryer basket.

Serve and enjoy.

Savory Dash Seasoned Pork Chops

Preparation Time: 10 minutes

Cooking Time: 20 minutes

Serve: 4

Ingredients:

4 pork chops, boneless

2 tbsp dash seasoning

Directions:

Coat pork chops with seasoning.

Select Air Fry mode.

Set time to 20 minutes and temperature 360 F then press START.

The air fryer display will prompt you to ADD FOOD once the temperature is reached then place pork chops in the air fryer basket.

Turn pork chops halfway through.

Serve and enjoy.

Spicy Asian Lamb

Preparation Time: 10 minutes

Cooking Time: 10 minutes

Serve: 4

Ingredients:

1 lb lamb, cut into 2-inch pieces

1 tbsp soy sauce

2 tbsp vegetable oil

1/2 tsp cayenne

1 1/2 tbsp ground cumin

1/4 tsp liquid stevia

2 red chili peppers, chopped

1 tbsp garlic, minced

1 tsp salt

Directions:

Mix together cumin and cayenne in a small bowl.

Rub meat with cumin mixture and place in a large bowl.

Add oil, soy sauce, garlic, chili peppers, stevia, and salt over the meat.

Mix well and place in the refrigerator overnight.

Select Air Fry mode.

Set time to 10 minutes and temperature 360 F then press START.

The air fryer display will prompt you to ADD FOOD once the temperature is reached then place marinated meat in the air fryer basket.

Serve and enjoy.

Chipotle Steak

Preparation Time: 10 minutes

Cooking Time: 10 minutes

Serve: 3

Ingredients:

1 lb ribeye steak

1/4 tsp onion powder

1/4 tsp garlic powder

1/4 tsp chili powder

1/2 tsp black pepper

1/2 tsp coffee powder

1/8 tsp cocoa powder

1/8 tsp coriander powder

1/4 tsp chipotle powder

1/4 tsp paprika

1 1/2 tsp sea salt

Directions:

In a small bowl, mix together all ingredients except steak.

Rub spice mixture all over the steak and let sit the steak for 30 minutes.

Select Air Fry mode.

Set time to 10 minutes and temperature 390 F then press START.

The air fryer display will prompt you to ADD FOOD once the temperature is reached then place steak in the air fryer basket.

Turn steak halfway through. Serve and enjoy.

Baked Lamb Chops

Preparation Time: 10 minutes

Cooking Time: 20 minutes

Serve: 5

Ingredients:

5 lamb rib chops

1 garlic clove, grated

2 tbsp olive oil 1 tsp paprika

1/2 tsp smoked paprika

1 tsp cumin

1/2 tbsp

 oregano

Directions:

In a small bowl, mix together paprika, smoked paprika, cumin, oregano, garlic, and 1 tbsp olive oil.

Coat lamb chops with spice mixture and place in the refrigerator for 3 hours.

Heat remaining 1 tbsp olive oil in a pan over medium-high heat.

Once the oil is hot then place lamb chops and cook for 3 minutes or until browned.

Select Bake mode.

Set time to 16 minutes and temperature 375 F then press START.

The air fryer display will prompt you to ADD FOOD once the temperature is reached then place lamb chops in the air fryer basket.

Turn lamb chops halfway through.

Serve and enjoy.

Lemon Garlic Sirloin Steak

Preparation Time: 10 minutes

Cooking Time: 30 minutes

Serve: 6

Ingredients:

2 lbs sirloin steak, cut into 1-inch pieces

2 garlic cloves, minced

1 1/2 cups fresh parsley, chopped

1/2 tsp black pepper

3 tbsp fresh lemon juice

1 tsp dried oregano

1/4 cup water

1/4 cup olive oil

1 tsp salt

Directions:

Add all ingredients except beef into the large bowl and mix well together.

Pour bowl mixture into the large zip-lock bag.

Add beef into the bag and shake well and refrigerate for 1 hour.

Select Bake mode.

Set time to 30 minutes and temperature 400 F then press START.

The air fryer display will prompt you to ADD FOOD once the temperature is reached then place marinated beef in the air fryer basket.

Serve and enjoy.

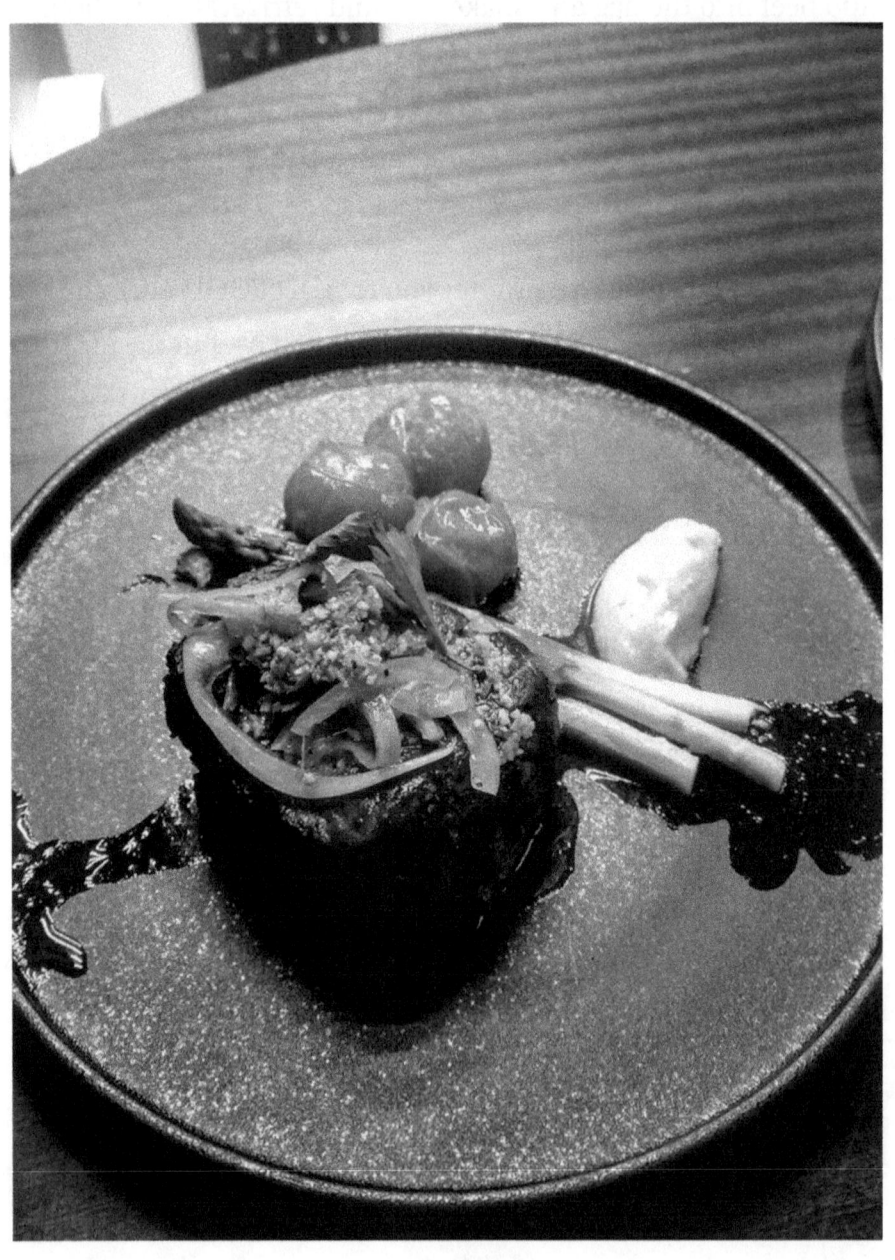

www.ingramcontent.com/pod-product-compliance
Lightning Source LLC
Chambersburg PA
CBHW071110030426
42336CB00013BA/2027